Keto Vegetarian Recipes for Beginners

Lose Weight and Improve Your Health with These Easy Plant-Based Ketogenic Diet Recipes

Lidia Wong

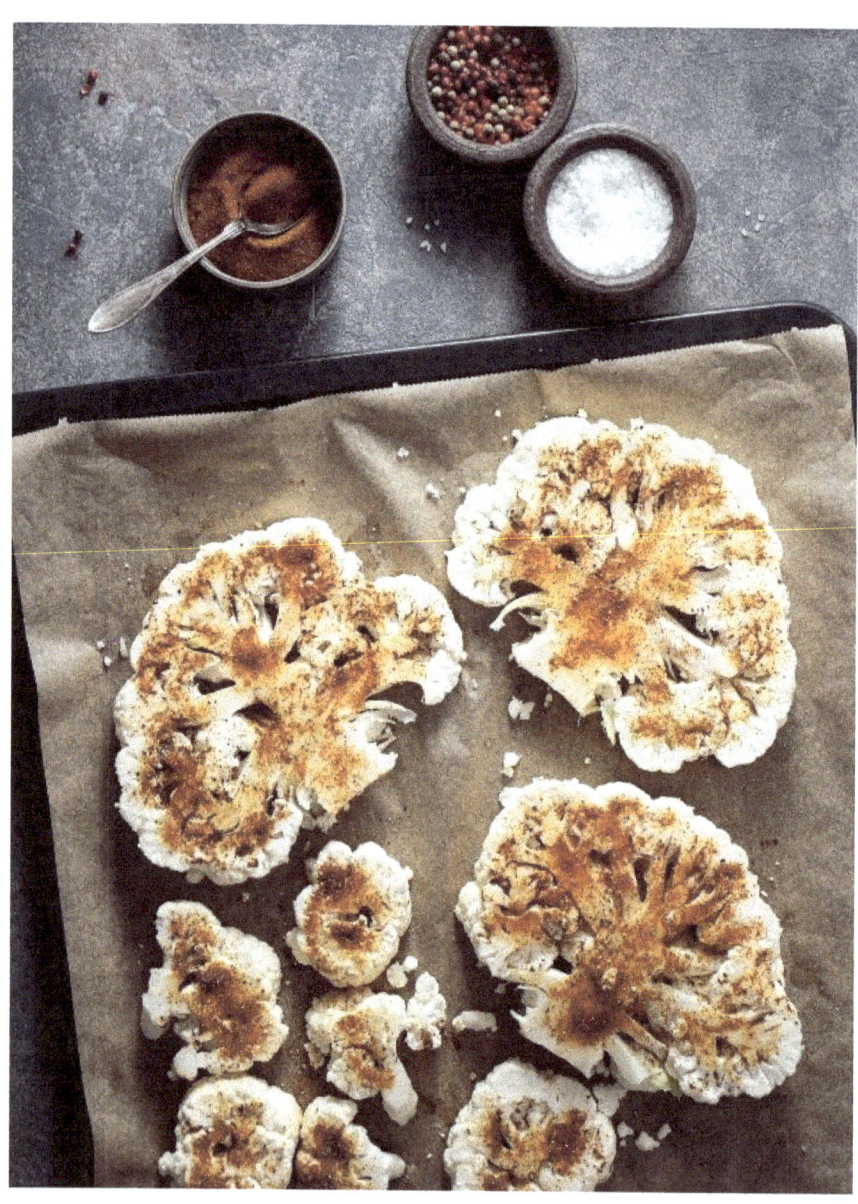

© **Copyright 2021 by Lidia Wong - All rights reserved.**

The content contained within this book may not be reproduced, duplicated or transmitted without direct written permission from the author or the publisher.
Under no circumstances will any blame or legal responsibility be held against the publisher, or author, for any damages, reparation, or monetary loss due to the information contained within this book. Either directly or indirectly.

Legal Notice:
This book is copyright protected. This book is only for personal use. You cannot amend, distribute, sell, use, quote or paraphrase any part, or the content within this book, without the consent of the author or publisher.

Disclaimer Notice:
Please note the information contained within this document is for educational and entertainment purposes only. All effort has been executed to present accurate, up to date, and reliable, complete information. No warranties of any kind are declared or implied. Readers acknowledge that the author is not engaging in the rendering of legal, financial, medical or professional advice. The content within this book has been derived from various sources. Please consult a licensed professional before attempting any techniques outlined in this book.
By reading this document, the reader agrees that under no circumstances is the author responsible for any losses, direct or indirect, which are incurred as a result of the use of information contained within this document, including, but not limited to, — errors, omissions, or inaccuracies.

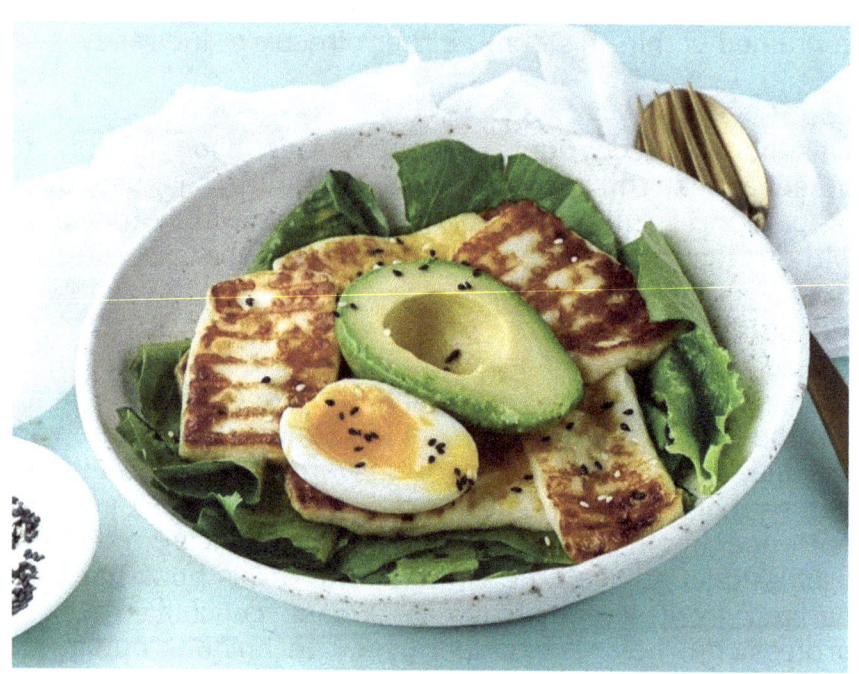

TABLE OF CONTENTS

INTRODUCTION 1

Keto Zucchini Fritters 3

Gouda Breakfast Soufflés 5

Eggplant and Olives Stew 7

Greens and Vinaigrette 9

Mustard Greens and Kale Mix 10

Sweet Kale and Onions Mix 12

Italian Bok Choy, Rice and Arugula Salad 13

Baked Zucchini Eggplant with Cheese 15

Keto Tofu and Spinach Casserole 17

Healthy Braised Garlic Kale 19

Tomatoes and Eggs Plate 21

Cauliflower And Broccoli Side Dish 23

Peppers Rice 25

Orange Scallions and Brussels Sprouts 27

Glazed Curried Carrots 29

Eggplant Mix 31

Hearty Baby Carrots 33

Sensitive Steamed Artichokes 35

Zucchini Cakes	37
Hot & Sour Tofu Soup	39
Quick Thai Coconut Mushroom Soup	41
Garlic-Butter Tempeh with Shirataki Fettucine	43
Eggplant Ragu	45
Keto Vegan Bacon Carbonara	47
Black Bean Taco Salad Bowl	50
Moroccan Aubergine Salad	53
Sesame Cucumber Salad	55
Asian Slaw	57
Darn Good Caesar Salad	59
Pear and Arugula Salad	61
Refried Bean And Salsa Quesadillas	63
Tempeh Tantrum Burgers	65
Sesame- Wonton Crisps	67
Turmeric Peppers Platter	69
Absolute Avocado Pizza	70
Chocolate Melt Chaffles	72
Strawberry Shortcake Chaffle Bowls	74
Easy Keto Bread	76
Roasted Almonds	78
Almond Fat Bombs	80

Raspberry Protein Shake (vegan) 82

Pecan and Date-Stuffed Roasted Pears 84

Fruit Salad 86

Chocolate Watermelon Cups 87

Blueberry Brownies. 88

Rice and Cantaloupe Ramekins 90

Berries and Cherries Bowls 92

Nuts and Seeds Pudding 93

Cocoa Berries Mousse 95

Cold Grapes and Avocado Cream 96

Walnuts and Coconut Cake 97

Dates Cream 99

NOTE **101**

INTRODUCTION

The keto diet is the shortened term for ketogenic diet and it is essentially a high-fat and low-carb diet that helps you lose weight, thereby bringing various health benefits. This diet drastically restricts your carb intake while increasing your fat intake; this pushes your body to go into a state know as "*ketosis*". We will tackle ketosis in a bit.

The human body uses glucose from carbs to fuel metabolic pathways—meaning various bodily functions like digestion, breathing, etc.. Essentially, anything that needs energy. Even when you are resting, the body needs fuel or energy for you to continue living. If you think about it, when have you ever stopped breathing, or your heart stopped beating, or your liver stopped from cleansing the body, or your kidneys from filtering blood?

Never, unless you're dead, which is the only time in which the body doesn't need energy. In normal circumstances, glucose is the primary pathway when it comes to sourcing the body's energy.

But the body also has another pathway; it can utilize fats to fuel the various bodily processes. And this is what we call "*ketosis*". And the body can only enter ketosis when there is no glucose available, thus the reason for sticking to a low-carb diet is essential in the keto diet. Since no glucose is available, the body is pushed to use fats—it can either come from the food you consume or from your body's fat reserves—the adipose tissue or from the flabby parts of your body. This is how the keto diet helps you lose weight, by burning up all those stored fats that you have and using it to fuel bodily processes.

That said, if for whatever reason you are a vegetarian, following a ketogenic diet can be extremely difficult. A vegetarian diet is largely free of animal products, which means that food tends to be usually high in carbohydrates. Still, with careful planning, it is possible. This Cookbook will provide you with various easy and delicious dishes to help you stick to your ketogenic diet plan while being a vegetarian.

Enjoy!

Keto Zucchini Fritters

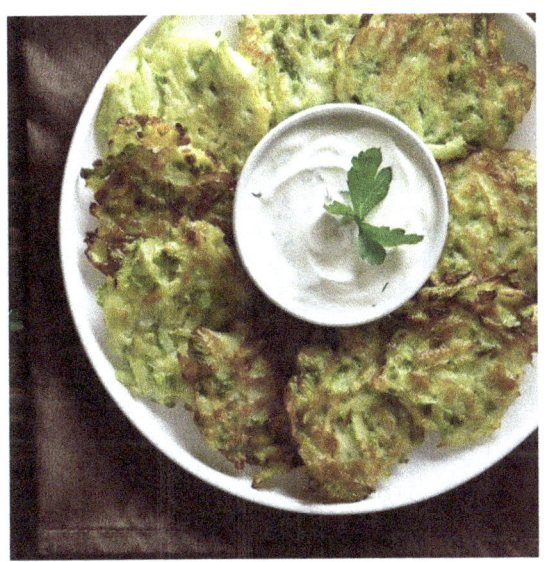

Preparation Time: 25 minutes

Cooking Time: 6 minutes

Servings: 8

Ingredients:

- 2 organic eggs
- 1 lb. zucchini, grated and squeezed
- 1 teaspoon salt
- 1 ½ ounces onion, minced
- 1 teaspoon lemon pepper

- ½ cup almond flour
- ½ teaspoon baking powder
- ¼ coconut flour
- ¼ cup Parmesan cheese, grated

Directions:

1. Add your zucchini, eggs, and onion in a mixing bowl and mix until well combined. Add all the remaining ingredients into another mixing bowl, and stir well. Add your dry ingredients to the zucchini mixture and mix well. Pour enough oil into the pan to cover the bottom surface of it. Heat the oil over medium-high heat. Once the oil becomes hot, pour ¼ cup zucchini batter into pan and cook for 3 minutes then flip and cook the other side for another 3 minutes. Place your fried zucchini fritters on a paper towel to soak up the excess oil. Serve and enjoy!

Nutritional Values (Per Serving):

Calories: 81 Fat: 6 g Carbohydrates: 5 g Sugar: 0 g Protein: 5 g Cholesterol: 58 mg

Gouda Breakfast Soufflés

Preparation Time: 10minutes

Cooking Time: 10minutes

Servings: 4

Ingredients:

- 2 ½ tbsp butter, softened
- 2 ½ tbsp almond flour
- 4 yolks, beaten
- 1 ½ tsp mustard powder
- ½ cup almond milk
- 2 ½ cup Gouda cheese, grated + a little extra for topping
- 2 egg whites, beaten until stiff

Directions:

1. Preheat the oven to 375 °F and lightly brush the inner parts of four medium ramekins with ½ tablespoon of butter.
2. Melt the remaining 2 tablespoons of butter in a small pan over low heat and stir in the almond flour, cook for 1 minute, stirring constantly.

Remove from the heat, mix in the mustard powder until evenly combined and slowly whisk in the milk until no lumps form.
3. Return to medium heat, while still stirring until the sauce comes to a rolling boil. Stir in the cheese until melted. Turn the heat off.
4. Into the egg yolks whisk ¼ cup of the warmed milk mixture, then combine with the remaining milk sauce. Fold in the egg whites gradually until evenly combined.
5. Spoon the mixture into the ramekins and top with the remaining cheese. Bake in the oven for 8 to 10 minutes or until the soufflés have a slight wobble, but soft at the center.
6. Allow cooling for 5 minutes and serve.

Nutrition:

Calories: 570, Total Fat: 57.6g, Saturated Fat: 35.5g, Total Carbs: 12 g, Dietary Fiber: 5g, Sugar: 3g, Protein: 10g, Sodium: 814mg

Eggplant and Olives Stew

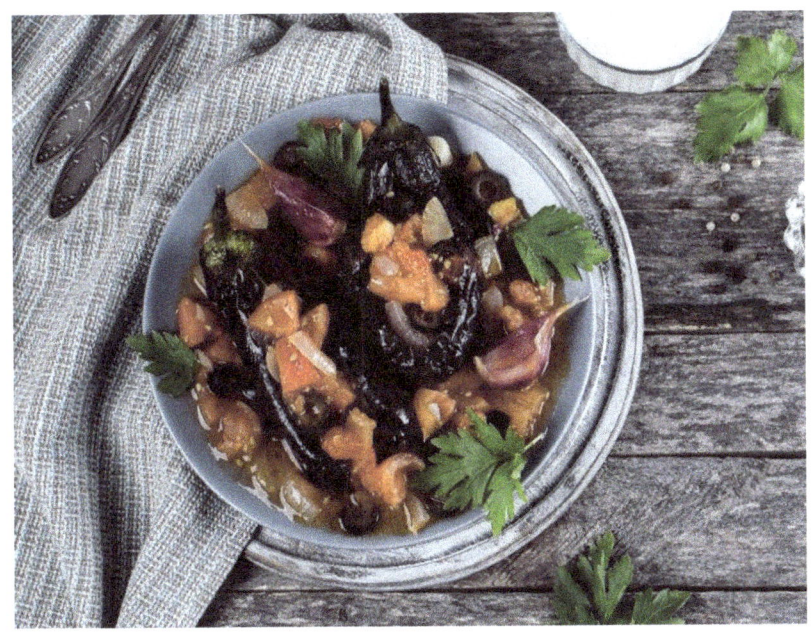

Preparation time: 10 minutes

Cooking time: 30 minutes

Servings: 4

Ingredients:

- 2 scallions, chopped
- 2 tablespoons avocado oil
- 2 garlic cloves, chopped
- 1 bunch parsley, chopped

- 1 teaspoon basil, dried
- 1 teaspoon cumin, dried
- Salt and black pepper to the taste
- 2 eggplants, roughly cubed
- 1 cup green olives, pitted and sliced
- 3 tablespoons balsamic vinegar
- ½ cup tomato passata

Directions:

1. Heat up a pot with the oil over medium heat, add the scallions, garlic, basil and cumin and sauté for 5 minutes.
2. Add the eggplants and the other ingredients, toss, cook over medium heat for 25 minutes more, divide into bowls and serve.

Nutrition:

Calories 93, fat 1.8, fiber 10.6, carbs 18.6, protein 3.4

Greens and Vinaigrette

Preparation time: 10 minutes

Cooking time: 0 minutes

Servings: 4

Ingredients:

- 1 cup baby kale
- 1 cup baby arugula
- 1 cup romaine lettuce
- 1 cucumber, cubed
- 3 tablespoons lime juice
- 2 tomatoes, cubed
- 1/3 cup olive oil
- 1 tablespoon balsamic vinegar
- Salt and black pepper to the taste

Directions:

1. In a bowl, combine the oil with the vinegar, lime juice, salt and pepper and whisk well.
2. In another bowl, combine the greens with the vinaigrette, toss and serve right away.

Nutrition:

Calories 112, fat 9, fiber 2, carbs 6, protein 2

Mustard Greens and Kale Mix

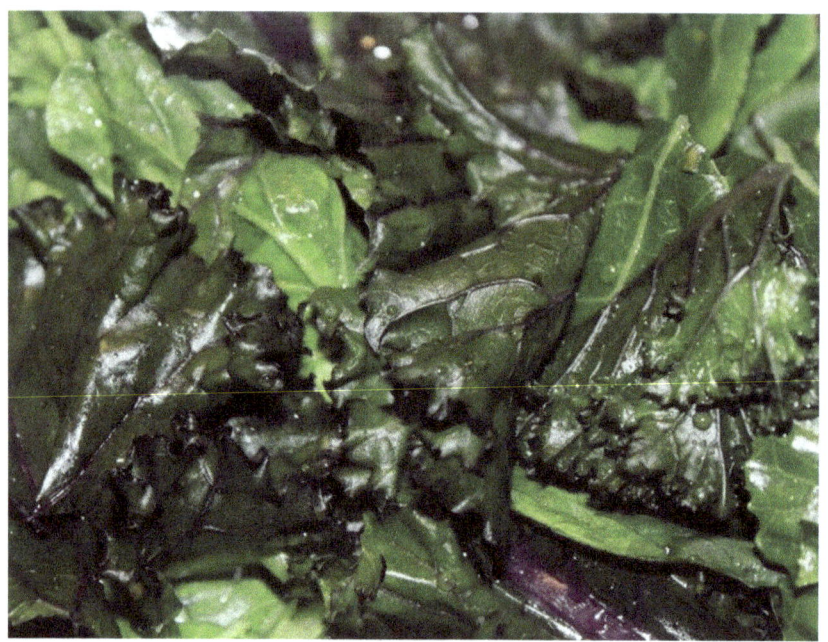

Preparation time: 10 minutes

Cooking time: 10 minutes

Servings: 4

Ingredients:

- ½ pound kale, torn
- 1 pound mustard greens
- 2 celery stalks, chopped

- 2 tablespoons avocado oil
- 1 cup tomatoes, cubed
- 2 avocados, peeled, pitted and cubed
- 1 cup coconut cream
- 2 tablespoons lemon juice
- 2 garlic cloves minced
- 2 tablespoons parsley, chopped
- A pinch of salt and black pepper

Directions:

1. Heat up a pan with the oil over medium heat, add the mustard greens, kale, celery and the other ingredients, toss, cook for 10 minutes, divide between plates and serve warm.

Nutrition:

Calories 200, fat 4, fiber 8, carbs 16, protein 7

Sweet Kale and Onions Mix

Preparation time: 10 minutes

Cooking time: 12 minutes

Servings: 4

Ingredients:

- 4 cups kale, torn
- 4 spring onions, chopped
- ½ cup tomato passata
- 2 tablespoons avocado oil
- A pinch of sea salt and black pepper
- 1 teaspoon stevia
- 1 teaspoon sweet paprika

Directions:

1. Heat up a pan with the oil over medium-high heat, add the spring onions, paprika and stevia, toss and cook for 2 minutes.
2. Add the kale and the other ingredients, toss, cook over medium heat for 10 minutes, divide between plates and serve right away.

Nutrition:

Calories 150, fat 4, fiber 4, carbs 8.2, protein 5

Italian Bok Choy, Rice and Arugula Salad

Preparation time: 10 minutes

Cooking time: 0 minutes

Servings: 4

Ingredients:

- 2 cups cauliflower rice, steamed
- 1 cup bok choy, torn
- 2 tomatoes, cubed
- ½ cup baby arugula
- 2 tablespoons pine nuts, toasted
- 1 tablespoon walnuts, chopped
- 2 tablespoons avocado oil
- 2 garlic cloves, minced
- 2 tablespoons basil, chopped
- 1 tablespoon Italian seasoning
- 2 tablespoons lime juice
- A pinch of sea salt and black pepper

Directions:

1. In a salad bowl, combine the cauliflower rice with the arugula, bok choy and the other ingredients, toss, divide into smaller bowls and serve.

Nutrition:

Calories 227, fat 2, fiber 7, carbs 18, protein 11

Baked Zucchini Eggplant with Cheese

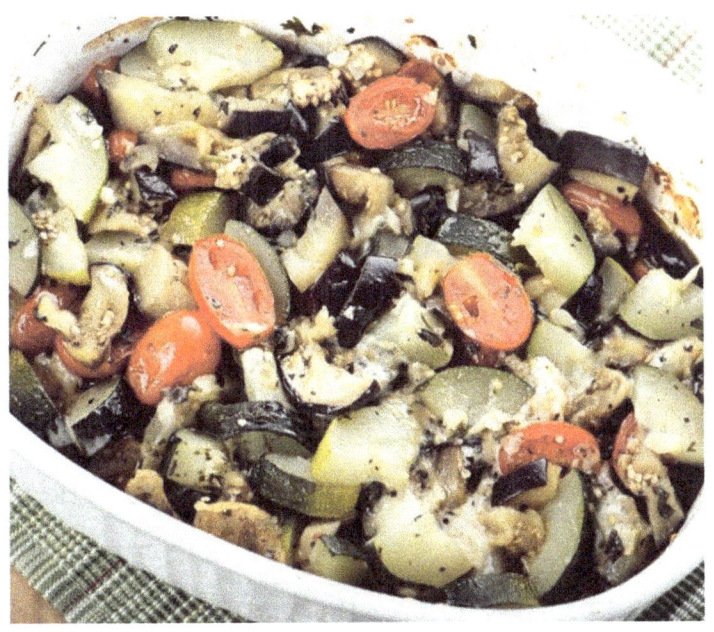

Preparation Time: 15 minutes

Cooking Time: 35 minutes

Servings: 6

Ingredients:

- 3 medium zucchinis, sliced
- 3-ounces Parmesan cheese, grated
- 1 tablespoon extra-virgin olive oil
- 1 medium eggplant, sliced

- 1 cup cherry tomatoes, halved
- ¼ cup basil, chopped
- ¼ cup parsley, chopped
- 4 garlic cloves, minced
- ¼ teaspoon sea salt
- ¼ teaspoon pepper

Directions:

1. Preheat your oven to 350°Fahrenheit. Spray a baking dish with cooking spray. In a mixing bowl, add eggplant, cherry tomatoes, zucchini, olive oil, cheese, basil, garlic, salt, and pepper, toss to mix. Transfer eggplant mixture to baking dish and place into a preheated oven to bake for 35 minutes. Garnish with chopped parsley. Serve and enjoy!

Nutritional Values (Per Serving):

Calories: 110 Cholesterol: 10 mg Carbohydrates: 10.4 g Fat: 5.8 g Sugar: 4.8 g Protein: 7 g

Keto Tofu and Spinach Casserole

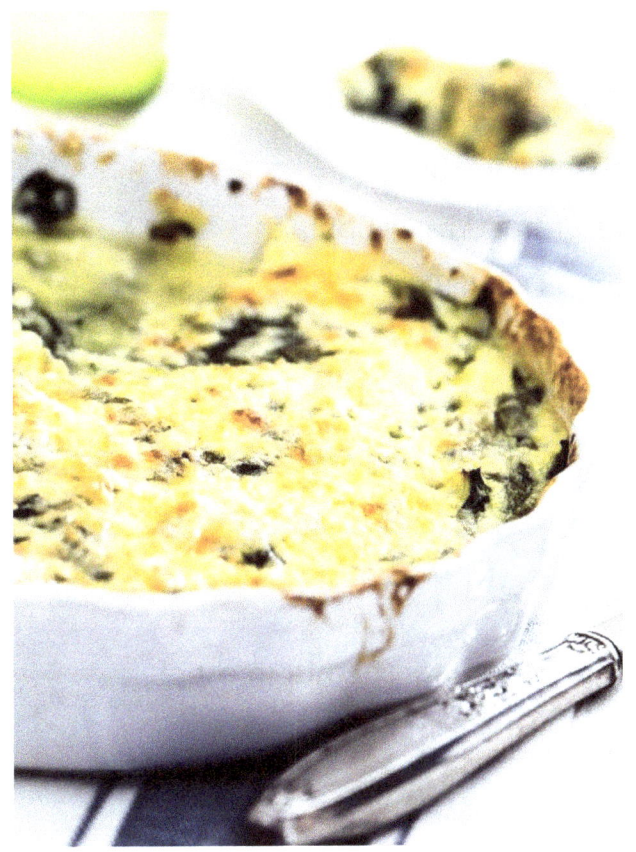

Preparation Time: 5 min

Cooking Time: 5 min

Serves: 4

Ingredients:

- 1 Bell Pepper, diced
- 1 block Firm Tofu, drained, pressed, and cut into cubes
- ½ White Onion, minced
- 2 tbsp Olive Oil
- 100 grams Fresh Spinach
- ½ cup Diced Tomatoes
- 1 tsp Paprika
- 1 tsp Garlic Powder
- Salt and Pepper to taste

Directions:

1. Combine all ingredients in a pot.
2. Simmer for 5 minutes

Nutritional Values:

Kcal per serve: 222 Fat: 15 g. Protein: 17 g. Carbs: 7 g.

Healthy Braised Garlic Kale

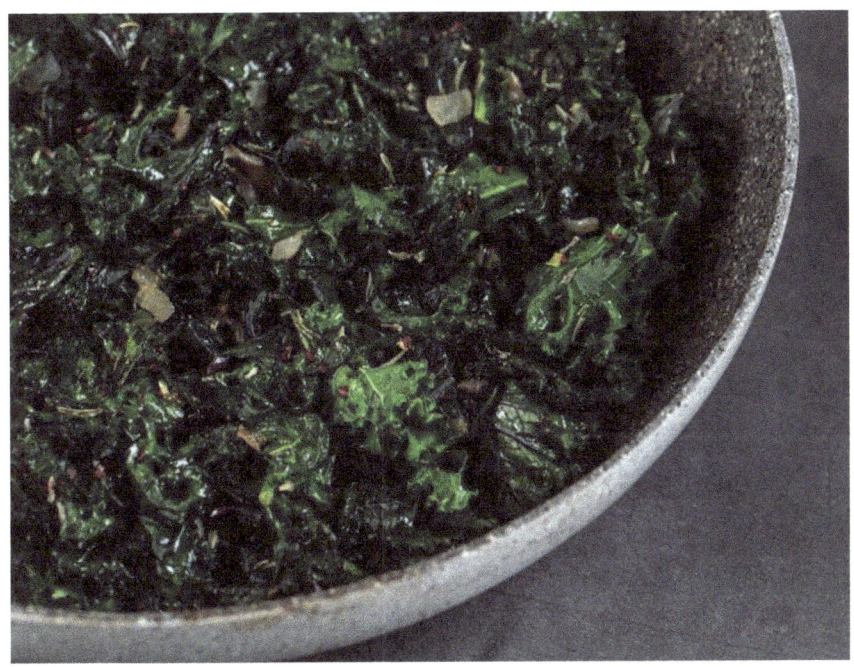

Preparation Time: 50 minutes

Servings: 4

Ingredients:

- 10 oz kale, stems removed and chopped
- 2 cups vegetable stock
- 1 tsp chili pepper flakes, dried
- 4 tbsp coconut oil

- 1 medium onion, sliced
- 4 garlic cloves, minced
- 1 tsp sea salt

Directions:

1. Heat coconut oil in a pan over medium heat.
2. Once the oil is hot then add onion, garlic and chili pepper flakes and sauté until lightly brown.
3. Pour vegetable stock and stir well.
4. Now add chopped kale and season with salt. Stir well.
5. Cover pan with lid and cook on low heat for 40 minutes.
6. Serve and enjoy.

Nutritional Value (Amount per Serving):

Calories 172 Fat 14 g Carbohydrates 11 g Sugar 1 g Protein 2 g Cholesterol 0 mg

Tomatoes and Eggs Plate

Preparation Time: 10 minutes

Cooking Time: 17 minutes

Serving: 4

Ingredients:

- 8 eggs
- 5 oz vegan bacon, chopped
- 1 tbsp olive oil
- Salt and black pepper to taste
- 1 tbsp butter, room temperature
- ¼ cup red cherry tomatoes
- 2 tbsp chopped fresh oregano

Directions:

1. Cook the vegan bacon in a medium skillet over medium heat until brown and crispy, 5 minutes. Divide onto 4 plates and set aside.
2. Add half of the olive oil into the skillet to heat and crack 4 eggs into the oil. Cook until the egg whites set, but the yolk still runny, 1 minute. Spoon two eggs to the side of the vegan bacon

in two plates and fry the remaining eggs using the remaining olive oil. Plate the eggs on two more plates.
3. Melt the butter in the same skillet, cook in the tomatoes until brown around the edges and a bit on the skin, 8 minutes. Add the egg plates.
4. Season the food with salt, black pepper, and garnish with the oregano.
5. Serve warm.

Nutrition:

Calories: 501, Total Fat:43.3 g, Saturated Fat: 21.5g, Total Carbs: 17 g, Dietary Fiber: 5g, Sugar: 7g, Protein18: g, Sodium: 656mg

Cauliflower And Broccoli Side Dish

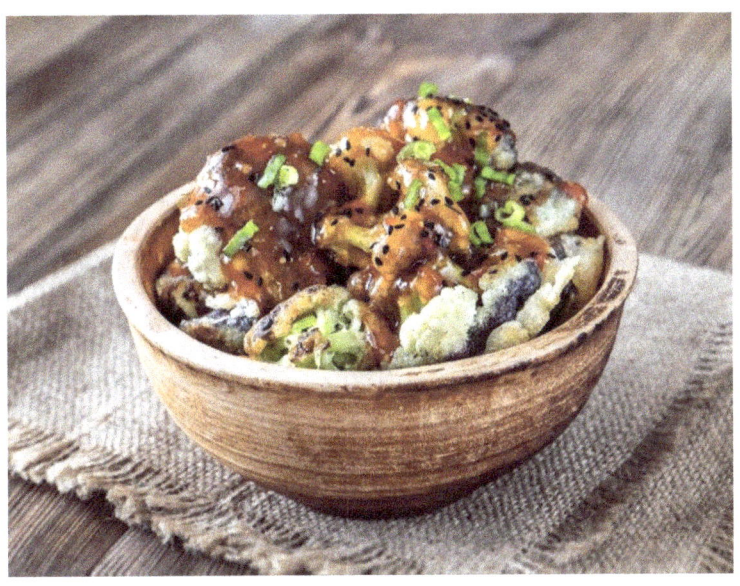

Preparation time: 10 minutes

Cooking time: 3 hours

Servings: 10

Ingredients:

- 4 cups broccoli florets
- 14 ounces tomato paste
- 4 cups cauliflower florets
- 1 yellow onion, chopped
- 1 teaspoon thyme, dried

- Salt and black pepper to the taste
- ½ cup almonds, sliced

Directions:

1. In your slow cooker, mix broccoli with cauliflower, tomato paste, onion, thyme, salt and pepper, toss, cover and cook on High for 3 hours.
2. Add almonds, toss, divide between plates and serve as a side dish.
3. Enjoy!

Nutrition:

Calories 177, fat 12, fiber 2, carbs 10, protein 7

Peppers Rice

Preparation time: 10 minutes

Cooking time: 25 minutes

Servings: 4

Ingredients:

- 1 yellow bell pepper, chopped
- 1 red bell pepper, chopped
- 1 green bell pepper, chopped
- 4 scallions, chopped
- 2 cups cauliflower rice
- 1 cup vegetable stock
- 1 tablespoon olive oil
- 1 teaspoon coriander, ground
- 1 teaspoon cumin, ground
- 1 teaspoon basil, dried
- 1 teaspoon oregano, dried
- 1 tablespoon chives, chopped
- A pinch of salt and black pepper

Directions:

1. Heat up a pan with the oil over medium heat, add the scallions and the peppers and sauté for 5 minutes.
2. Add the cauliflower rice and the other ingredients, toss, cook over medium heat for 20 minutes, divide between plates and serve as a side dish.

Nutrition:

Calories 69, fat 4.4, fiber 1.3, carbs 8.9, protein 1.3

Orange Scallions and Brussels Sprouts

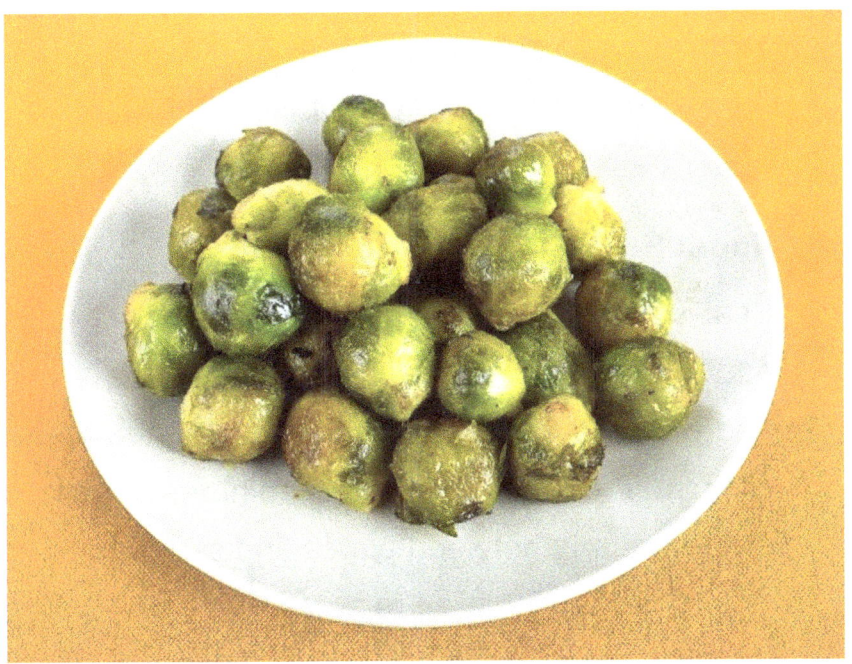

Preparation time: 10 minutes

Cooking time: 25 minutes

Servings: 4

Ingredients:

- 1 pound Brussels sprouts, trimmed and halved
- 1 cup scallions, chopped

- Zest of 1 lime, grated
- 1 tablespoon olive oil
- ¼ cup orange juice
- 2 tablespoons stevia
- A pinch of salt and black pepper

Directions:

1. Heat up a pan with the oil over medium heat, add the scallions and sauté for 5 minutes.
2. Add the sprouts and the other ingredients, toss, cook over medium heat for 20 minutes more, divide the mix between plates and serve.

Nutrition:

Calories 193, fat 4, fiber 1, carbs 8, protein 10

Glazed Curried Carrots

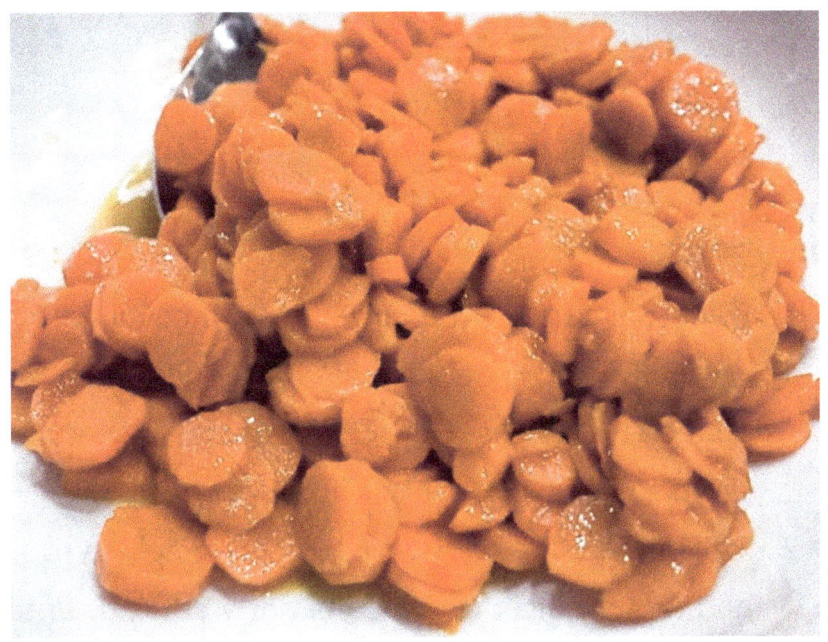

Preparation time: 5 minutes

cooking time: 15 minutes

servings: 6

Ingredients

- 1 pound carrots, peeled and thinly sliced
- 2 tablespoons olive oil

- juice of ½ lemon
- 2 tablespoons curry powder
- 2 tablespoons pure maple syrup
- sea salt
- freshly ground black pepper

Directions

1. Place the carrots in a large pot and cover with water. Cook on medium-high heat until tender, about 10 minutes. Drain the carrots and return them to the pan over medium-low heat.
2. Stir in the olive oil, curry powder, maple syrup, and lemon juice. Cook, constantly stirring, until the liquid reduces, about 5 minutes. Season with salt and pepper and serve immediately.

Eggplant Mix

Preparation time: 10 minutes

Cooking time: 40 minutes

Servings: 3

Ingredients:

- 5 medium eggplants, sliced into rounds
- 1 teaspoon thyme, chopped
- 2 tablespoons balsamic vinegar
- 1 teaspoon mustard
- ½ cup olive oil
- 2 garlic cloves, minced
- Black pepper to taste
- A pinch of sea salt
- 1 teaspoon maple syrup

Directions:

1. In a bowl, mix vinegar with thyme, mustard, garlic, oil, salt, pepper and maple syrup and whisk very well.

2. Arrange eggplant round on a lined baking sheet, place in the oven at 425 degrees F and roast for 40 minutes.
3. Divide eggplants between plates and serve.
4. Enjoy!

Nutritional value/serving:

Calories 533, fat 35,6, fiber 32,6, carbs 56,5, protein 9,4

Hearty Baby Carrots

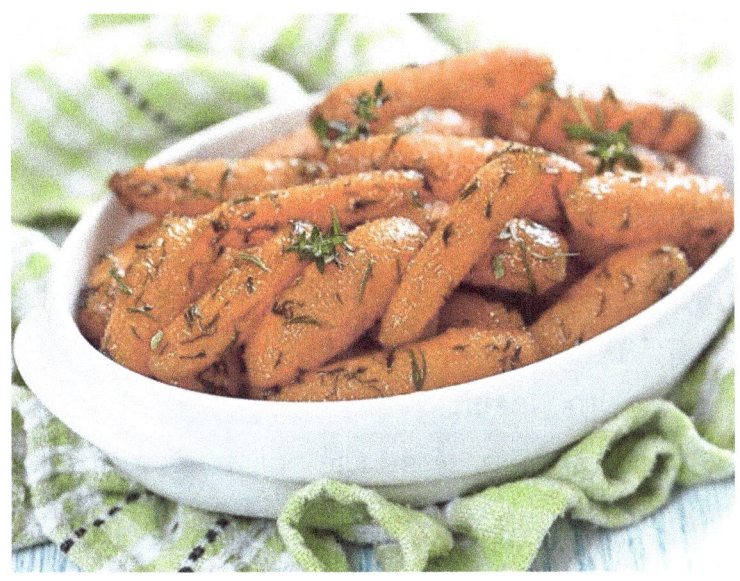

Preparation Time: 5 mins

Servings: 4

Ingredients:

- 1 tbsp. chopped fresh mint
- 1 c. water
- 1 lb. baby carrots
- Sea flavored vinegar
- 1 tbsp. clarified ghee

Directions:

1. Place a steamer rack on top of your pot and add the carrots
2. Add water
3. Lock up the lid and cook at HIGH pressure for 2 minutes
4. Do a quick release
5. Pass the carrots through a strainer and drain them
6. Wipe the insert clean
7. Return the insert to the pot and set the pot to Sauté mode
8. Add clarified butter and allow it to melt
9. Add mint and sauté for 30 seconds
10. Add carrots to the insert and sauté well
11. Remove them and sprinkle with bit of flavored vinegar on top
12. Enjoy!

Nutrition:

Calories: 131, Fat:10 g, Carbs:11 g, Protein:1 g, Sugars:5 g, Sodium:190 mg

Sensitive Steamed Artichokes

Preparation Time: 5 mins

Servings: 4

Ingredients:

- 1 halved lemon
- ¼ tsp. paprika
- 2 tbsps. Homemade Whole30 mayo
- 2 medium artichokes
- 1 tsp. Dijon mustard

Directions:

1. Wash the artichokes and remove the damaged outer leaves
2. Trim the spines and cut off upper edge
3. Wipe the cur edges with lemon half
4. Slice the stem and peel the stem
5. Chop it up and keep them on the side
6. Add a cup of water to the pot and place a steamer basket inside

7. Transfer the artichokes to the steamer basket and a squeeze of lemon
8. Lock up the lid and cook on HIGH pressure for 10 minutes
9. Release the pressure naturally
10. Enjoy

Nutrition:

Calories: 77, Fat:5 g, Carbs:0 g, Protein:2 g, Sugars:1.3 g, Sodium:121 mg

Zucchini Cakes

Preparation Time: 10 mins

Servings: 4

Ingredients:

- Freshly ground black pepper
- 1 finely diced red onion
- 2 tsps. Salt
- 1 egg white
- 1 shredded medium zucchini
- ¾ c. salt-free breadcrumbs
- Homemade horseradish sauce

Directions:

1. Preheat oven to 400 °F. Spray a baking sheet lightly with oil and set aside.
2. Press shredded zucchini gently between paper towels to remove excess liquid.
3. In a large bowl, combine zucchini, onion, egg white, breadcrumbs, seasoning, and black pepper. Mix well.

4. Shape mixture into patties and place on the prepared baking sheet.
5. Place baking sheet on middle rack in oven and bake for 10 minutes. Gently flip patties and return to oven to bake for another 10 minutes.
6. Remove from oven and serve immediately.

Nutrition:

Calories: 94, Fat:1 g, Carbs:19 g, Protein:4 g, Sugars:31 g, Sodium:161 mg

Hot & Sour Tofu Soup

Preparation Time: 40 Minutes

Cooking Time: 15 Minutes

Servings:3

Ingredients

- 6 to 7 ounces firm or extra-firm tofu
- 1 teaspoon olive oil
- 1 cup sliced mushrooms
- 1 cup finely chopped cabbage
- 1 garlic clove, minced
- 4 cups water or Economical Vegetable Broth
- ½-inch piece fresh ginger, peeled and minced
- 2 tablespoons rice vinegar or apple cider vinegar
- 2 tablespoons soy sauce
- 1 teaspoon toasted sesame oil
- 1 teaspoon sugar
- Pinch red pepper flakes
- Salt
- 1 scallion, white and light green parts only, chopped

Directions

1. Preparing the Ingredients.
2. Press your tofu before you start: Put it between several layers of paper towels and place a heavy pan or book (with a waterproof cover or protected with plastic wrap) on top. Let stand for 30 minutes. Discard the paper towels. Cut the tofu into ½-inch cubes.
3. In a large soup pot, heat the olive oil over medium-high heat.
4. Add the mushrooms, cabbage, garlic, ginger, and a pinch of salt. Sauté for 7 to 8 minutes, until the vegetables are softened.
5. Add the water, vinegar, soy sauce, sesame oil, sugar, red pepper flakes, and tofu.
6. Bring to a boil, then turn the heat to low. Simmer the soup for 5 to 10 minutes.
7. Serve with the scallion sprinkled on top.
8. Leftovers will keep in an airtight container for up to 1 week in the refrigerator or up to 1 month in the freezer.

Nutrition Per Serving (2 cups)

Calories: 161; Protein: 13g; Total fat: 9g; Saturated fat: 1g; Carbohydrates: 10g; Fiber: 3g

Quick Thai Coconut Mushroom Soup

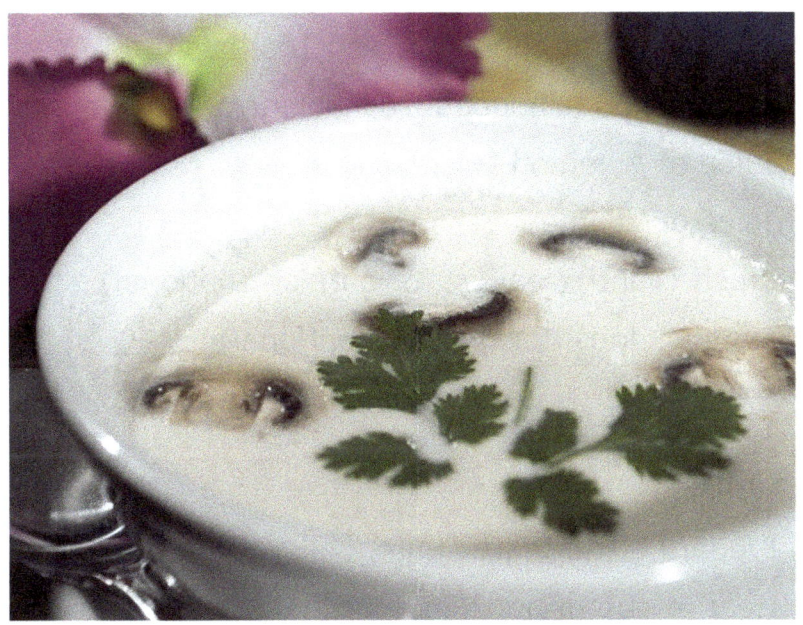

Preparation Time: 5 Minutes

Cooking Time: 10 Minutes

Servings: 4

Ingredients

- 1½ cups low-sodium vegetable broth, divided
- 1 tablespoon minced fresh ginger
- 2 garlic cloves, minced

- 1 (8-ounce) package baby bella or white button mushrooms, stemmed and sliced
- 1 (13.5-ounce) can full-fat coconut milk
- 2 tablespoons chopped fresh Thai basil
- 1 tablespoon chopped fresh cilantro
- Juice of ½ lemon
- Juice of ½ lime
- Fresh cilantro leaves, for garnish (optional)
- Lime wedges, for garnish (optional)

Directions

1. Preparing the Ingredients.
2. Heat ½ cup of broth in a large saucepot over medium-high heat. Sauté the garlic and ginger in the broth for 1 minute, or until fragrant.
3. Add the mushrooms and slowly pour in the remaining 1 cup of broth. Bring to a boil and reduce the heat to a simmer. Add the coconut milk, lemon juice, lime juice, basil, and chopped cilantro.
4. Let simmer for 5 minutes, or until heated through. Garnish with whole cilantro leaves and lime wedges, if desired.

Garlic-Butter Tempeh with Shirataki Fettucine

Preparation Time: 30 minutes

Serving: 4

Ingredients:

For the shirataki fettuccine:

- 2 (8 oz) packs shirataki fettuccine

For the garlic-butter steak bites:

- 4 tbsp butter
- 1 lb thick-cut tempeh, cut into 1-inch cubes
- 4 garlic cloves, mined
- 2 tbsp chopped fresh parsley
- Salt and black pepper to taste
- 1 cup freshly grated parmesan cheese

Directions:

For the shirataki fettuccine:

1. Boil 2 cups of water in a medium pot over medium heat.
2. Strain the shirataki pasta through a colander and rinse very well under hot running water.

3. Allow proper draining and pour the shirataki pasta into the boiling water. Cook for 3 minutes and strain again.
4. Place a dry skillet over medium heat and stir-fry the shirataki pasta until visibly dry, and makes a squeaky sound when stirred, 1 to 2 minutes. Take off the heat and set aside.

For the garlic-butter mushroom bites:

5. Melt the butter in a large skillet, season the mushroom with salt, black pepper and cook in the butter until brown, and cooked through, 10 minutes.
6. Stir in the garlic and cook until fragrant, 1 minute.
7. Mix in the parsley and shirataki pasta; toss well and season with salt and black pepper.
8. Dish the food, top with the parmesan cheese and serve immediately.

Nutrition:

Calories:399, Total Fat: 34.2g, Saturated Fat: 18.6g, Total Carbs: 10 g, Dietary Fiber:0g, Sugar: 2g, Protein:17 g, Sodium: 283mg

Eggplant Ragu

Preparation Time: 20 minutes

Serving: 4

Ingredients

- 1 lb eggplant
- 2 tbsp butter
- 1/4 cup sugar-free tomato sauce
- 4 tbsp chopped fresh parsley + extra for garnishing
- 4 large green bell peppers, Blade A, noodles trimmed
- Salt and black pepper to taste
- 4 large red bell peppers, Blade A, noodles trimmed
- 1 small red onion, Blade A, noodles trimmed
- 1 cup grated parmesan cheese

Directions:

1. Heat half of the butter in a medium skillet and cook the eggplant until brown, 5 minutes. Season with salt and black pepper.

2. Stir in the tomato sauce, parsley, and cook for 10 minutes or until the sauce reduces by a quarter.
3. Stir in the bell pepper and onion noodles; cook for 1 minute and turn the heat off.
4. Adjust the taste with salt, black pepper, and dish the food onto serving plates.
5. Garnish with the parmesan cheese and more parsley; serve warm.

Nutrition:

Calories: 163, Total Fat: 9.8g, Saturated Fat:5.6 g, Total Carbs: 7 g, Dietary Fiber:2g, Sugar:4g, Protein: 13g, Sodium: 417mg

Keto Vegan Bacon Carbonara

Preparation Time: 30 minutes + overnight chilling time

Serving size: 4

Ingredients:

For the keto pasta:

- 1 cup shredded mozzarella cheese
- 1 large egg yolk

For the carbonara:

- 4 egg yolks
- 4 vegan bacon slices, chopped
- 1¼ cups coconut whipping cream
- ¼ cup mayonnaise
- Salt and black pepper to taste
- 1 cup grated parmesan cheese + more for garnishing

Directions:

For the pasta:

1. Pour the cheese into a medium safe-microwave bowl and melt in the microwave for 35 minutes

or until melted.
2. Take out the bowl and allow cooling for 1 minute only to warm the cheese but not cool completely. Mix in the egg yolk until well combined.
3. Lay a parchment paper on a flat surface, pour the cheese mixture on top and cover with another parchment paper. Using a rolling pin, flatten the dough into 1/8-inch thickness.
4. Take off the parchment paper and cut the dough into thin spaghetti strands. Place in a bowl and refrigerate overnight.
5. When ready to cook, bring 2 cups of water to a boil in a medium saucepan and add the pasta.
6. Cook for 40 seconds to 1 minute and then drain through a colander. Run cold water over the pasta and set it aside to cool.

For the carbonara:

7. Add the vegan bacon to a medium skillet and cook over medium heat until crispy, 5 minutes. Set aside.
8. Pour the coconut whipping cream into a large pot and allow simmering for 3 to 5 minutes.
9. Whisk in the mayonnaise and season with the

salt and black pepper. Cook for 1 minute and spoon 2 tablespoons of the mixture into a medium bowl. Allow cooling and mix in the egg yolks.
10. Pour the mixture into the pot and mix quickly until well combined. Stir in the parmesan cheese to melt and fold in the pasta.
11. Spoon the mixture into serving bowls and garnish with more parmesan cheese. Cook for 1 minute to warm the pasta.
12. Serve immediately.

Nutrition:

Calories:456, Total Fat: 38.2g, Saturated Fat:14.7g, Total Carbs:13 g, Dietary Fiber:3g, Sugar: 8g, Protein:16g, Sodium:604 mg

Black Bean Taco Salad Bowl

Preparation time: 15 minutes

cooking time: 5 minutes

servings: 3

Ingredients

For the black bean salad

- 1 (14-ouncecan black beans, drained and rinsed, or 1½ cups cooked
- 1 cup corn kernels, fresh and blanched, or frozen and thawed
- ¼ cup fresh cilantro, or parsley, chopped
- Zest and juice of 1 lime
- 1 to 2 teaspoons chili powder
- Pinch sea salt
- 1½ cups cherry tomatoes, halved
- 1 red bell pepper, seeded and chopped
- 2 scallions, chopped

For 1 serving of tortilla chips

- 1 large whole-grain tortilla or wrap
- 1 teaspoon olive oil
- Pinch sea salt

- Pinch freshly ground black pepper
- Pinch dried oregano
- Pinch chili powder

For 1 bowl

- 1 cup fresh greens (lettuce, spinach, or whatever you like
- ¼ cup Fresh Mango Salsa
- ¾ cup cooked quinoa, or brown rice, millet, or other whole grain
- ¼ cup chopped avocado, or Guacamole

Directions

To Make The Black Bean Salad

1. Toss All The Ingredients Together In A Large Bowl.
2. To Make The Tortilla Chips
3. Brush The Tortilla With Olive Oil, Then Sprinkle With Salt, Pepper, Oregano, Chili Powder, And Any Other Seasonings You Like. Slice It Into Eighths Like A Pizza.
4. Transfer The Tortilla Pieces To A Small Baking Sheet Lined With Parchment Paper And Put In The Oven Or Toaster Oven To Toast Or Broil For 3 To 5 Minutes, Until Browned. Keep An Eye On

Them, As They Can Go From Just Barely Done To Burned Very Quickly.

To Make The Bowl

5. Lay The Greens In The Bowl, Top With The Cooked Quinoa, ⅓ Of The Black Bean Salad, The Avocado, And Salsa.

Nutrition:

Calories: 589; Total fat: 14g; Carbs: 101g; Fiber: 20g; Protein: 21g

Moroccan Aubergine Salad

Preparation time: 30 minutes

cooking time: 15 minutes

servings: 2

Ingredients

- 1 teaspoon olive oil
- 1 eggplant, diced
- ¼ teaspoon ground nutmeg
- Pinch sea salt
- ½ teaspoon ground cumin
- ½ teaspoon ground ginger
- ¼ teaspoon turmeric
- 1 lemon, half zested and juiced, half cut into wedges
- 2 tablespoons capers
- 1 tablespoon chopped green olives
- 1 garlic clove, pressed
- Handful fresh mint, finely chopped
- 2 cups spinach, chopped

Directions

1. Heat the oil in a large skillet on medium heat, then sauté the eggplant. Once it has softened slightly, about 5 minutes, stir in the cumin, ginger, turmeric, nutmeg, and salt. Cook until the eggplant is very soft, about 10 minutes.
2. Add the lemon zest and juice, capers, olives, garlic, and mint. Sauté for another minute or two, to blend the flavors. Put a handful of spinach on each plate, and spoon the eggplant mixture on top.
3. Serve with a wedge of lemon, to squeeze the fresh juice over the greens.
4. To tenderize the eggplant and reduce some of its naturally occurring bitter taste, you can sweat the eggplant by salting it. After dicing the eggplant, sprinkle it with salt and let it sit in a colander for about 30 minutes. Rinse the eggplant to remove the salt, then continue with the recipe as written.

Nutrition

Calories: 97; Total fat: 4g; Carbs: 16g; Fiber: 8g; Protein: 4g

Sesame Cucumber Salad

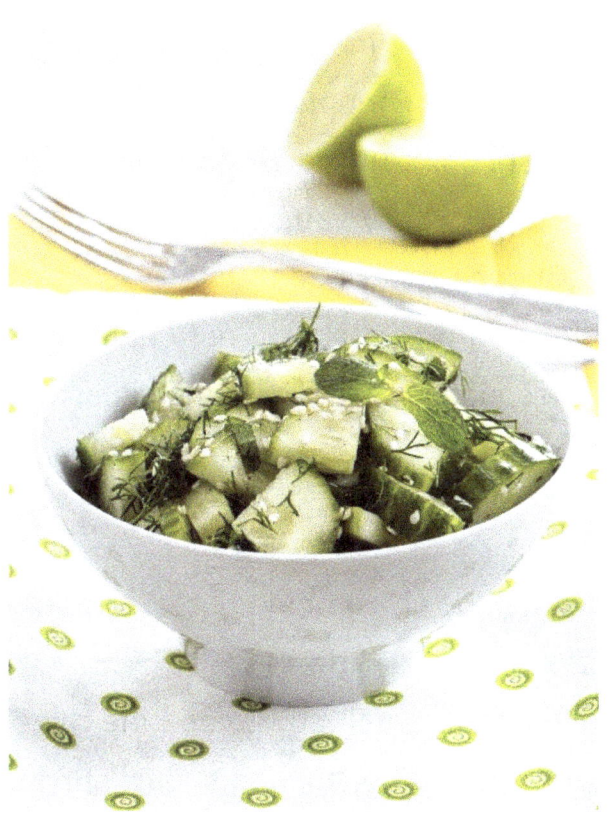

Preparation time: 15 minutes

cooking time: 0 minutes

servings: 4 to 6

Ingredients

- 2 medium English cucumbers, peeled and cut into 1/4-inch slices
- 1 tablespoon mirin
- 2 tablespoons chopped fresh parsley
- 3 tablespoons toasted sesame oil
- 2 tablespoons soy sauce
- 2 teaspoons rice vinegar
- 1 teaspoon brown sugar (optional
- 2 tablespoons toasted sesame seeds

Directions

1. In a small bowl, combine the cucumbers and parsley and set aside.
2. In a separate small bowl, combine the oil, soy sauce, mirin, vinegar, and sugar, stirring to blend. Pour the dressing over the cucumbers. Set aside for at least 10 minutes.
3. Spoon the cucumber salad into small bowls, sprinkle with sesame seeds, and serve.

Asian Slaw

Preparation Time: 15 Minutes

Cooking Time: 0 Minutes

Servings:4

Ingredients

- 8 ounces napa cabbage, cut crosswise into 1/4-inch strips
- 1 cup grated carrot
- 1 cup grated daikon radish
- 2 green onions, minced
- 1 tablespoon soy sauce
- 1 teaspoon grated fresh ginger
- 2 tablespoons chopped fresh parsley
- 2 tablespoons rice vinegar
- 1 tablespoon grapeseed oil
- 2 teaspoons toasted sesame oil
- 1/2 teaspoon dry mustard
- Salt and freshly ground black pepper
- 2 tablespoons chopped unsalted roasted peanuts, for garnish (optional)

Directions

1. In a large bowl, combine the napa cabbage, carrot, daikon, green onions, and parsley. Set aside.
2. In a small bowl, combine the vinegar, grapeseed oil, sesame oil, soy sauce, ginger, mustard, and salt and pepper to taste. Stir until well blended. Pour the dressing over the vegetables and toss gently to coat. Taste, adjusting seasonings if necessary. Cover and refrigerate to allow flavors to blend, about 2 hours. Sprinkle with peanuts, if using, and serve.

Darn Good Caesar Salad

Preparation Time: 10 Minutes

Cooking Time: 0 Minutes

Servings:4

Ingredients

For The Dressing

- ½ cup walnuts
- ½ cup water
- Juice of ½ lime
- 3 tablespoons olive oil
- 1 tablespoon white miso paste
- 1 teaspoon soy sauce or gluten-free tamari
- 1 teaspoon Dijon mustard
- 1 teaspoon garlic powder
- ¼ teaspoon sea salt
- ½ teaspoon black pepper

For The Salad

- 2 heads romaine lettuce, chopped
- 1 cup cherry tomatoes, halved
- Walnut Parmesan or store-bought vegan Parmesan, for garnish

- Vegan croutons, for garnish (optional)

Directions

1. To make the dressing: In a blender, combine all the dressing ingredients and blend until almost smooth, about 2 minutes. It's okay if this dressing is slightly chunky, which is more like a classic Caesar dressing texture.
2. To make the salad: In a large bowl, toss the lettuce with half of the dressing. Add more as desired. Divide among serving plates and top with the tomatoes and Parmesan. Finish the salad off with croutons, if desired.

Pear and Arugula Salad

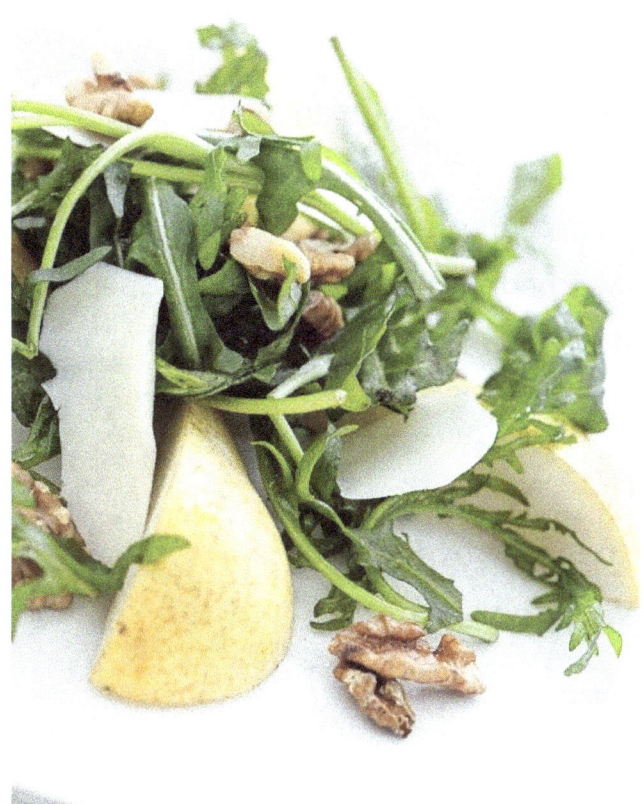

Preparation Time: 10 Minutes

Cooking Time: 8 Minutes

Servings:4

Ingredients

- 10 ounces arugula
- ¼ cup chopped pecans
- 2 pears, thinly sliced
- 1 tablespoon finely minced shallot
- 2 tablespoons champagne vinegar
- 2 tablespoons olive oil
- ¼ teaspoon sea salt
- ¼ teaspoon freshly ground black pepper
- ¼ teaspoon dijon mustard

Directions

1. Preheat the oven to 350°F.
2. Spread the pecans in a single layer on a baking sheet. Toast in the preheated oven until fragrant, about 6 minutes. Remove from the oven and let cool. In a large bowl, toss the pecans, arugula, and pears. In a small bowl, whisk together the shallot, vinegar, olive oil, salt, pepper, and -mustard. Toss with the salad and serve immediately.

Refried Bean And Salsa Quesadillas

Preparation time: 5 minutes

cooking time: 6 minutes

servings: 4 quesadillas

Ingredients

- 1 tablespoon canola oil, plus more for frying
- 11/2 cups cooked or 1 (15.5-ouncecan pinto beans, drained and mashed
- 4 (10-inchwhole-wheat flour tortillas
- 1 teaspoon chili powder
- 1 cup tomato salsa, homemade or store-bought
- 1/2 cup minced red onion (optional)

Directions

1. In a medium saucepan, heat the oil over medium heat. Add the mashed beans and chili powder and cook, stirring, until hot, about 5 minutes. Set aside.

2. To assemble, place 1 tortilla on a work surface and spoon about 1/4 cup of the beans across the bottom half. Top the beans with the salsa and onion, if using. Fold top half of the tortilla over the filling and press slightly.
3. In large skillet heat a thin layer of oil over medium heat. Place folded quesadillas, 1 or 2 at a time, into the hot skillet and heat until hot, turning once, about 1 minute per side.
4. Cut quesadillas into 3 or 4 wedges and arrange on plates. Serve immediately.

Tempeh Tantrum Burgers

Preparation time: 15 minutes

cooking time: 0 minutes

servings: 4 burgers

Ingredients

- 8 ounces tempeh, cut into 1/2-inch dice
- ¾ cup chopped onion
- 2 garlic cloves, chopped
- ¾ cup chopped walnuts
- 1/2 cup old-fashioned or quick-cooking oats
- 1 tablespoon minced fresh parsley
- 1/2 teaspoon dried oregano
- 1/2 teaspoon dried thyme
- 1/4 teaspoon freshly ground black pepper
- 1/2 teaspoon salt
- 3 tablespoons olive oil
- Dijon mustard
- 4 whole grain burger rolls
- Sliced red onion, tomato, lettuce, and avocado

Directions

1. In a medium saucepan of simmering water, cook the tempeh for 30 minutes. Drain and set aside to cool.
2. In a food processor, combine the onion and garlic and process until minced. Add the cooled tempeh, walnuts, oats, parsley, oregano, thyme, salt, and pepper. Process until well blended. Shape the mixture into 4 equal patties.
3. In a large skillet, heat the oil over medium heat. Add the burgers and cook until cooked thoroughly and browned on both sides, about 7 minutes per side.
4. Spread desired amount of mustard onto each half of the rolls and layer each roll with lettuce, tomato, red onion, and avocado, as desired. Serve immediately.

Sesame- Wonton Crisps

Preparation time: 10 minutes

cooking time: 10 minutes

servings: 12 crisps

Ingredients

- 12 Vegan Wonton Wrappers
- 2 tablespoons toasted sesame oil
- 12 shiitake mushrooms, lightly rinsed, patted dry, stemmed, and cut into 1/4-inch slices
- 4 snow peas, trimmed and cut crosswise into thin slivers
- 1 tablespoon fresh lime juice
- 1/2 teaspoon brown sugar
- 1 teaspoon soy sauce
- 1 medium carrot, shredded
- Toasted sesame seeds or black sesame seeds, if available

Directions

1. Preheat the oven to 350 °F. Lightly oil a baking sheet and set it aside. Brush the wonton wrappers with 1 tablespoon of the sesame oil and arrange on the baking sheet. Bake until golden brown and crisp, about 5 minutes. Set aside to cool. (Alternately, you can tuck the wonton wrappers into mini-muffin tins to create cups for the filling. Brush with sesame oil and bake them until crisp.
2. In a large skillet, heat the extra olive oil over medium heat. Add the mushrooms and cook until softened, 3 to 5 minutes. Stir in the snow peas and the soy sauce and cook 30 seconds. Set aside to cool.
3. In a large bowl, combine the lime juice, sugar, and remaining 1 tablespoon sesame oil. Stir in the carrot and cooled shiitake mixture. Top each wonton crisp with a spoonful of the shiitake mixture. Sprinkle with sesame seeds and arrange on a platter to serve.

Turmeric Peppers Platter

Preparation time: 10 minutes

Cooking time: 20 minutes

Servings: 4

Ingredients:

- 2 green bell peppers, cut into wedges
- 2 red bell peppers, cut into wedges
- 2 yellow bell peppers, cut into wedges
- 2 tablespoons avocado oil
- 2 garlic cloves, minced
- 1 bunch basil, chopped
- A pinch of salt and black pepper
- 2 tablespoons balsamic vinegar

Directions:

1. Heat up a pan with the oil over medium heat, add the garlic and the vinegar and cook for 2 minutes.
2. Add the peppers and the other ingredients, toss, cook over medium heat for 18 minutes, arrange them on a platter and serve as an appetizer.

Nutrition:

Calories 120, fat 8.2, fiber 2, carbs 4, protein 2.3

Absolute Avocado Pizza

Preparation Time: 10 minutes

Cooking Time: 25 minutes

Servings: 4

Ingredients:

Dough

- 2 eggs
- 4 tbsps. grated Parmesan cheese
- 2 envelopes unflavored gelatin
- ½ c. unsweetened Greek yogurt
- 4 tbsps. water
- 3 tbsps. grass-fed butter
- Salt

Filling

- Cheese, mushrooms, avocado puree, chopped fresh parsley

Directions:

1. Preheat oven to 450 degrees F.

2. Place all ingredients in a blender (gelatin without dissolving and beat well.
3. Grease a parchment paper with butter and evenly distribute the dough.
4. Place dough in greased baking pan and bake about 15 minutes.
5. Remove pizza from the oven and spread evenly with avocado sauce.
6. Top with your favorite fillings and sprinkle with the cheese.
7. Bake for 5 -10 minutes.
8. Remove from oven, let rest for 5 minutes and slice.
9. Serve immediately.

Nutrition:

Calories: 65, Fat: 20.87g, Carbs: 1.22g, Protein: 18.27g

Chocolate Melt Chaffles

Preparation Time: 15 minutes

Cooking Time: 36 minutes

Servings: 4

Ingredients:

For the chaffles:

- 2 eggs, beaten
- ¼ cup finely grated Gruyere cheese
- 2 tbsp heavy cream
- 1 tbsp coconut flour
- 2 tsp vanilla extract
- 2 tbsp cream cheese, softened
- 3 tbsp unsweetened cocoa powder
- A pinch of salt

For the chocolate sauce:

- 1/3 cup + 1 tbsp heavy cream
- 1 ½ oz unsweetened baking chocolate, chopped
- 1 ½ tsp sugar-free maple syrup
- 1 ½ tsp vanilla extract

Directions:

For the chaffles:

1. Preheat the cast iron pan.
2. In a medium bowl, mix all the ingredients for the chaffles.
3. Open the iron and add a quarter of the mixture. Close and cook until crispy, 7 minutes.
4. Transfer the chaffle to a plate and make 3 more with the remaining batter.

For the chocolate sauce:

5. Pour the heavy cream into a saucepan and simmer over low heat, 3 minutes.
6. Turn the heat off and add the chocolate. Allow melting for a few minutes and stir until fully melted, 5 minutes.
7. Mix in the maple syrup and vanilla extract.
8. Assemble the chaffles in layers with the chocolate sauce sandwiched between each layer.
9. Slice and serve immediately.

Nutrition:

Calories 172, Fats 13.57g, Carbs 6.65g, Net Carbs 3.65g, Protein 5.76g

Strawberry Shortcake Chaffle Bowls

Preparation Time: 10 minutes

Cooking Time: 28 minutes

Servings: 4

Ingredients:

- 1 egg, beaten
- ½ cup finely grated mozzarella cheese
- 1 tbsp almond flour
- 2 drops cake batter extract
- 1 cup cream cheese, softened
- 1 cup fresh strawberries, sliced
- 1 tbsp sugar-free maple syrup
- ¼ tsp baking powder

Directions:

1. Preheat the cast iron pan.
2. Meanwhile, in a medium bowl, whisk all the ingredients except the cream cheese and strawberries.

3. Open the iron, pour in half of the mixture, cover, and cook until crispy, 6 to 7 minutes.
4. Remove the chaffle bowl onto a plate and set aside.
5. Make a second chaffle bowl with the remaining batter.
6. To serve, divide the cream cheese into the chaffle bowls and top with the strawberries.
7. Drizzle the filling with the maple syrup and serve.

Nutrition:

Calories 235, Fats 20.62g, Carbs 5.9g, Net Carbs 5g, Protein 7.51g

Easy Keto Bread

Preparation time: 15 minutes

Cooking time: 1 hour & 15 minutes

Servings: 4

Ingredients:

- Nonstick cooking spray
- ¼ cup coconut flour
- 2 teaspoons baking powder
- 1 cup blanched almond flour
- ¼ teaspoon salt
- ⅓ cup coconut oil, melted
- 12 egg whites

Directions:

1. Preheat the oven to 350 °F. Spray a loaf pan with cooking spray, making sure to cover the interior corners and sides completely.
2. In the bowl of a food processor, combine the almond flour, coconut flour, baking powder, and salt. Pulse until well combined.
3. Add the coconut oil and pulse again until a crumble forms. Set aside.

4. In a large bowl, use a handheld electric mixer to beat the egg whites until stiff peaks form, about 10 minutes. (You can add ¼ teaspoon of cream of tartar to help the egg whites whip up faster.)
5. Add half the whipped egg whites to the food processor. Pulse a few times. Don't overbeat or you will deflate the egg whites.
6. Bit by bit, add the flour mixture to the remaining egg whites in the large bowl. Fold the flour into the egg whites very gently until well combined.
7. Spread the batter in the prepared bread pan.
8. Bake for 40 minutes, or until the top of the bread is lightly browned.
9. Place a layer of aluminum foil over the top of the bread (to avoid overbrowning) and cook for an additional 35 minutes.
10. Transfer the bread to a wire rack. When cooled, slice evenly.

Nutritions:

Calories 121, fat 9g, protein 5g, carbs 5g, fiber 3g, sugar 0g, sodium 86mg

Roasted Almonds

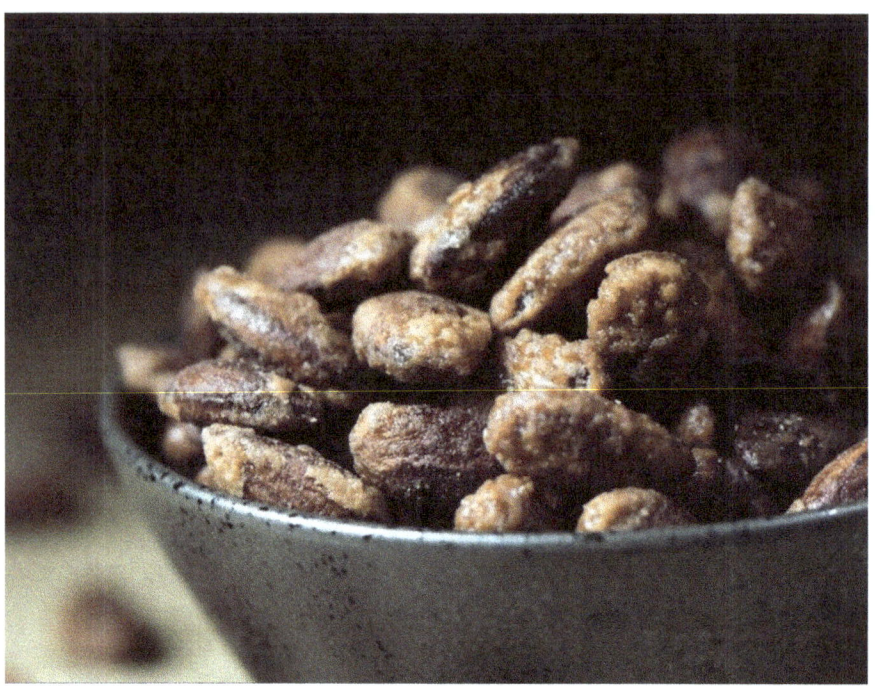

Preparation Time: 5 minutes

Cooking Time: 5 minutes

Servings: 4

Ingredients:

- 2 tablespoons rosemary
- 2 cups almonds, blanched

- 1 teaspoon salt
- 2 tablespoons olive oil
- 1 teaspoon paprika

Directions:

1. In a pan over medium-high heat add almonds and heat until toasted. Reduce heat to medium-low and add salt, paprika, and rosemary. Cook almonds for another 3 minutes. Serve immediately and enjoy!

Nutritions: (Per Servings):

Calories: 342 Fat: 31.1g Sugar: 2.1 g Carbohydrates: 11.5 g Cholesterol: 0 mg Protein: 10.2 g

Almond Fat Bombs

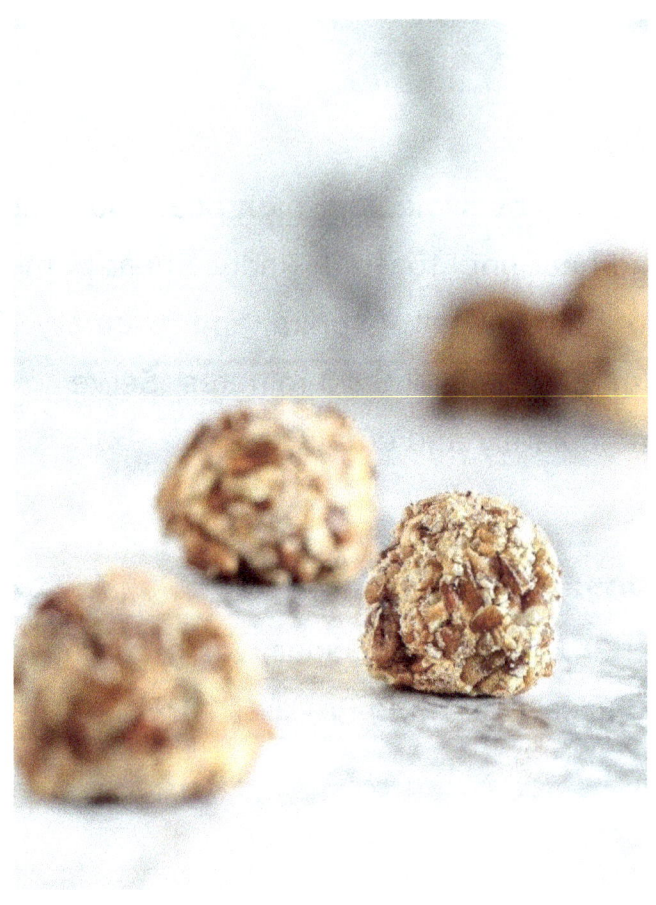

Preparation Time: 10 minutes

Cooking time: 25 minutes

Servings: 7

Ingredients:

- 1 cup almond flour
- ¼ cup coconut butter
- 2 tablespoon Erythritol
- 1 teaspoon vanilla extract
- 1 tablespoon almonds, crushed

Directions:

1. In the mixing bowl combine together almond flour and crushed almonds.
2. Add Erythritol, vanilla extract, and coconut butter.
3. Use the fork and knead the smooth and soft dough. Add more coconut butter if desired.
4. After this, make the medium size balls with the help of the fingertips and place them in the fridge for at least 25 minutes.
5. When the fat bombs are solid – they are cooked. Store the dessert in the fridge up to 5 days.

Nutritions:

Calories 156, fat 13.2, fiber 3.3, carbs 10, protein 4.2

Raspberry Protein Shake (vegan)

Preparation Time: 5 minutes

Cooking Time: 0 minute

Servings: 2

Ingredients:

- 1 cup full-fat coconut milk (or alternatively, use almond milk)
- 1 scoop organic soy protein (chocolate or vanilla flavor)
- ½ cup raspberries (fresh or frozen)
- 1 tbsp. low-carb maple syrup
- Optional: ¼ cup coconut cream
- Optional: 2-4 ice cubes

Directions:

1. Add all the ingredients to a blender, including the optional coconut cream and ice cubes if desired, and blend for 1 minute.
2. Transfer the shake to a large cup or shaker, and enjoy!

3. Alternatively, store the smoothie in an airtight container or a mason jar, keep it in the fridge, and consume within 2 days. Store for a maximum of 30 days in the freezer and thaw at room temperature.

Nutritions:

Calories: 311kcal, Net carbs: 4.6g, Fat: 25.7g, Protein: 14.65g, Fiber: 3.5g, Sugar: 3.35g

Pecan and Date-Stuffed Roasted Pears

Preparation time: 10 minutes

cooking time: 30 minutes

servings: 4

Ingredients

- 4 firm ripe pears, cored
- 1/2 cup finely chopped pecans
- 1 tablespoon fresh lemon juice
- 4 dates, pitted and chopped
- 1 tablespoon vegan margarine
- 1 tablespoon pure maple syrup
- 1/8 teaspoon ground ginger
- 1/4 teaspoon ground cinnamon
- 1/2 cup pear, white grape, or apple juice

Directions

1. Preheat the oven to 350 °F. Grease a shallow baking dish and set aside. Halve the pears lengthwise and use a melon baller to scoop out the cores. Rub the exposed part of the pears with the lemon juice to avoid discoloration.

2. In a medium bowl, combine the pecans, dates, margarine, maple syrup, cinnamon, and ginger and mix well.
3. Stuff the mixture into the centers of the pear halves and arrange them in the prepared baking pan. Pour the juice over the pears. Bake until tender, 30 to 40 minutes. Serve warm.

Fruit Salad

Preparation time: 2 hours

Cooking time: 0 minutes

Servings: 4

Ingredients:

- 2 avocados, peeled, pitted and cubed
- ½ cup strawberries, halved
- ½ cup blackberries
- ½ cup pineapple, peeled and cubed
- ¼ teaspoon vanilla extract
- 2 tablespoons stevia
- Juice of 1 lime

Directions:

- In a bowl, combine the avocados with the berries and the other ingredients, toss and keep in the fridge for 2 hours before serving.

Nutrition:

Calories 243, fat 22, fiber 0, carbs 6.2, protein 4

Chocolate Watermelon Cups

Preparation time: 2 hours

Cooking time: 0 minutes

Servings: 4

Ingredients:

- 2 cups watermelon, peeled and cubed
- 1 cup coconut cream
- 1 tablespoon stevia
- 1 tablespoon cocoa powder
- 1 tablespoon mint, chopped

Directions:

1. In a blender, combine the watermelon with the stevia and the other ingredients, pulse well, divide into cups and keep in the fridge for 2 hours before serving.

Nutrition:

Calories 164, fat 14.6, fiber 2.1, carbs 9.9, protein 2.1

Blueberry Brownies.

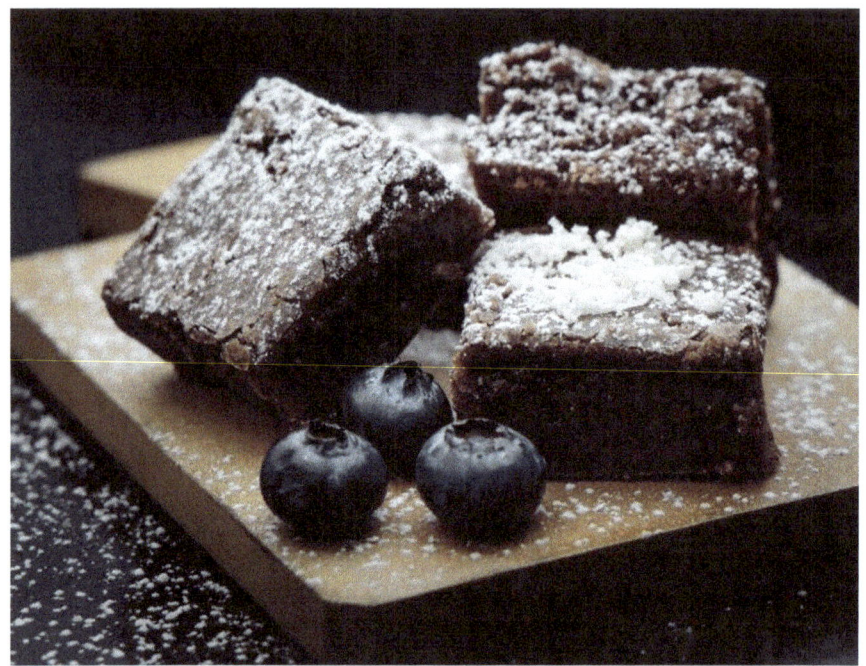

Preparation Time: 20 Minutes

Servings: 8

Ingredients:

- 1 cup cooked black beans
- ½ cup unsweetened cocoa powder
- ¾ cup unbleached all-purpose flour

- 1½ teaspoons baking powder
- 1 teaspoon pure vanilla extract
- ½ cup blueberry jam
- ½ cup natural sugar

Directions:

1. Lightly oil a baking tray that will fit in the steamer basket of your Cooker.
2. Blend together the beans, cocoa, jam, sugar, and vanilla.
3. Fold in the flour and baking powder until the batter is smooth.
4. Pour the batter into your tray and put the tray in your steamer basket.
5. Pour the minimum amount of water into the base of your Cooker and lower the steamer basket.
6. Seal and cook on Steam for 12 minutes.
7. Release the pressure quickly and set to one side to cool a little before slicing.

Rice and Cantaloupe Ramekins

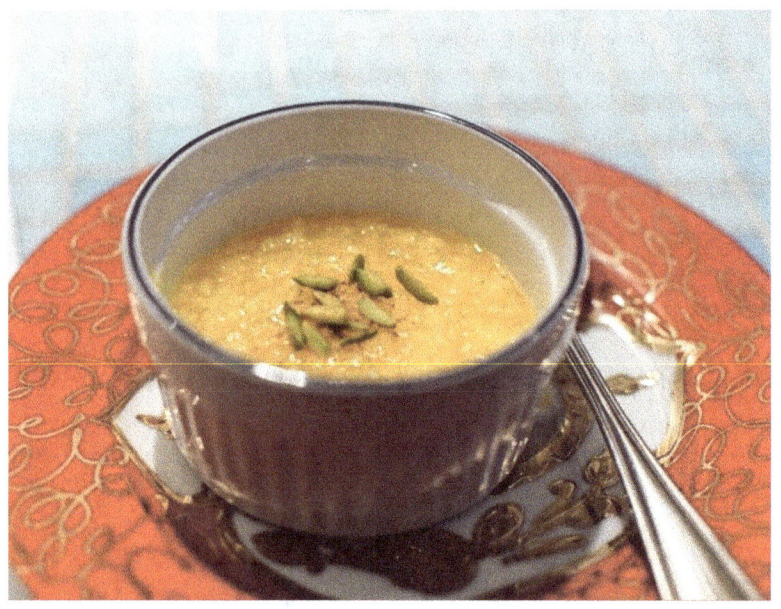

Preparation time: 10 minutes

Cooking time: 30 minutes

Servings: 4

Ingredients:

- 2 cups cauliflower rice, steamed
- 2 tablespoons flaxseed mixed with 3 tablespoons water

- ½ cup cantaloupe, peeled and chopped
- 1 cup coconut cream
- 2 tablespoons stevia
- 1 teaspoon vanilla extract
- Cooking spray

Directions:

1. In a bowl, mix the cauliflower rice with the flaxseed mix and the other ingredients except the cooking spray and whisk well.
2. Grease 4 ramekins with the cooking spray, divide the rice mix in each and cook at 360 degrees F for 30 minutes.
3. Serve cold.

Nutrition:

Calories 180, fat 5.3, fiber 5.4, carbs 11.5, protein 4

Berries and Cherries Bowls

Preparation time: 10 minutes

Cooking time: 0 minutes

Servings: 4

Ingredients:

- 1 cup strawberries, halved
- 1 cup blackberries
- 1 teaspoon vanilla extract
- 1 cup cherries, pitted and halved
- ¼ cup coconut cream
- ¼ cup stevia

Directions:

1. In a bowl, combine the berries with the cherries and the other ingredients, toss, divide into smaller bowls and serve cold.

Nutrition:

Calories 122, fat 4, fiber 5.3, carbs 6.6, protein 4.5

Nuts and Seeds Pudding

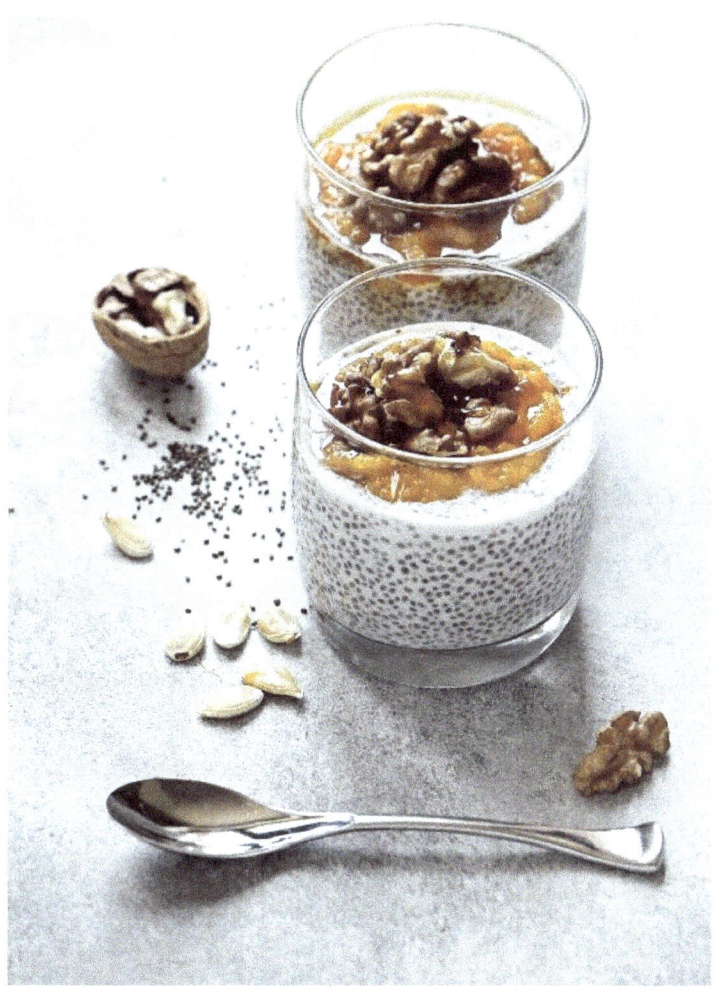

Preparation time: 10 minutes

Cooking time: 20 minutes

Servings: 4

Ingredients:

- 2 cups cauliflower rice
- ¼ cup coconut cream
- 2 cups almond milk
- 1 teaspoon vanilla extract
- 3 tablespoons stevia
- ½ cup walnuts, chopped
- 1 tablespoon chia seeds
- Cooking spray

Directions:

1. In a pan, combine the cauliflower rice with the cream, the almond milk and the other ingredients, toss, bring to a simmer and cook over medium heat for 20 minutes.
2. Divide into bowls and serve cold.

Nutrition:

Calories 223, fat 8.1, fiber 3.4, carbs 7.6, protein 3.4

Cocoa Berries Mousse

Preparation time: 10 minutes

Cooking time: 0 minutes

Servings: 2

Ingredients:

- 1 tablespoon cocoa powder
- ¾ cup coconut cream
- 1 cup blackberries
- 1 cup blueberries
- 1 tablespoon stevia

Directions:

1. In a blender, combine the berries with the cocoa and the other ingredients, pulse well, divide into bowls and keep in the fridge for 2 hours before serving.

Nutrition:

Calories 200, fat 8, fiber 3.4, carbs 7.6, protein 4.3

Cold Grapes and Avocado Cream

Preparation time: 1 hour

Cooking time: 0 minutes

Servings: 4

Ingredients:

- ½ cup stevia
- ½ cup coconut cream
- 2 cups grapes, halved
- 1 avocado, peeled, pitted and chopped
- 1 cup almond milk
- Zest of 1 lime, grated

Directions:

1. In a blender, combine the grapes with the avocado and the other ingredients, pulse well, divide into bowls and keep in the fridge for 1 hour before serving.

Nutrition:

Calories 152, fat 4.4, fiber 5.5, carbs 5.1, protein 0.8

Walnuts and Coconut Cake

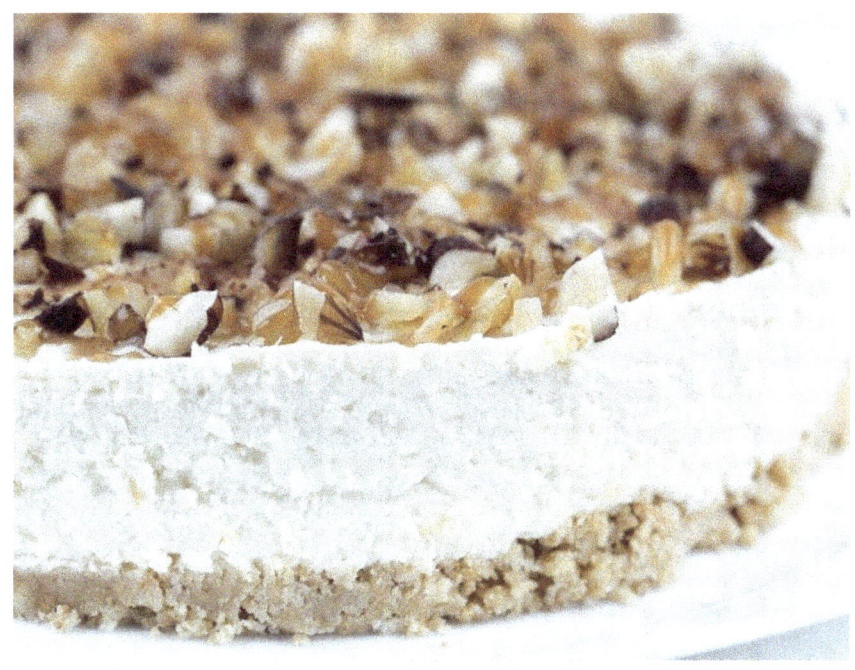

Preparation time: 10 minutes

Cooking time: 30 minutes

Servings: 8

Ingredients:

- 2 teaspoons baking powder
- 2 cups almond flour
- 1 cup avocado oil
- 1 cup coconut flesh, unsweetened and shredded

- 2 cups coconut milk
- 1 cup coconut cream
- 1 cup stevia
- 2 tablespoons walnuts, chopped
- 1 tablespoon lime juice
- 2 teaspoons vanilla extract
- Cooking spray

Directions:

1. In a bowl, mix the almond flour with the avocado oil, the coconut flesh, coconut milk and the other ingredients except for the cooking spray and whisk well.
2. Pour the mix into a cake pan greased with the cooking spray, introduce in the oven and bake at 370 degrees F for 30 minutes.
3. Leave the cake to cool down, cut and serve!

Nutrition:

Calories 200, fat 7.6, fiber 2.5, carbs 5.5, protein 4.5

Dates Cream

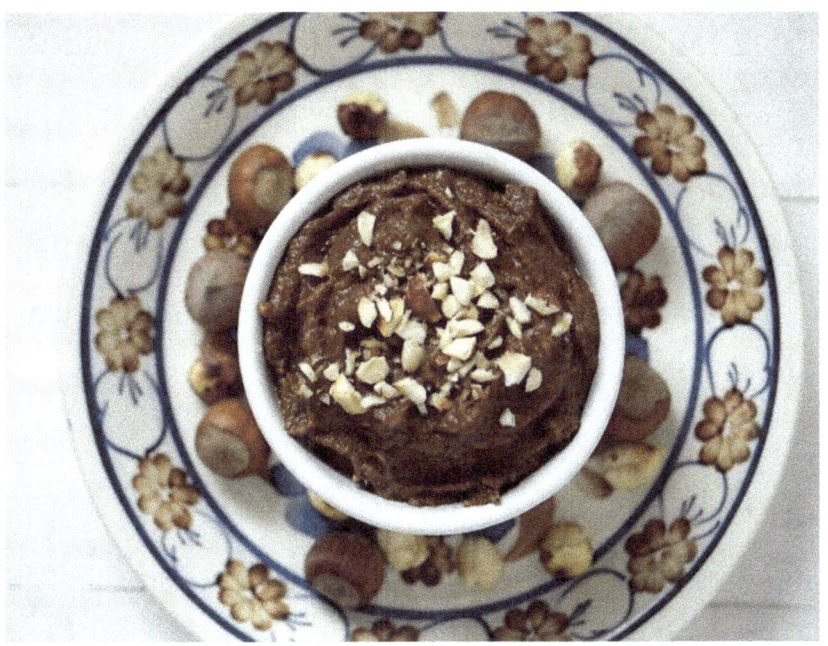

Preparation time: 10 minutes

Cooking time: 0 minutes

Servings: 2

Ingredients:

- 2 cups dates, chopped
- 1 cup coconut cream

- 2 tablespoons stevia
- ½ teaspoon nutmeg, ground
- 1 teaspoon vanilla extract
- 2 tablespoons water

Directions:

1. In a blender, combine the dates with the cream, the stevia and the other ingredients, pulse well, divide into cups and serve cold.

Nutrition:

Calories 192, fat 3.4, fiber 4.5, carbs 7.6, protein 3.5

NOTE

www.ingramcontent.com/pod-product-compliance
Lightning Source LLC
Chambersburg PA
CBHW070931080526
44589CB00013B/1481